OSTEOPOROSIS DIET COOKBOOK FOR SENIORS

Healthy and delicious recipes to help prevent bone loss and strengthen already weak bones at old age

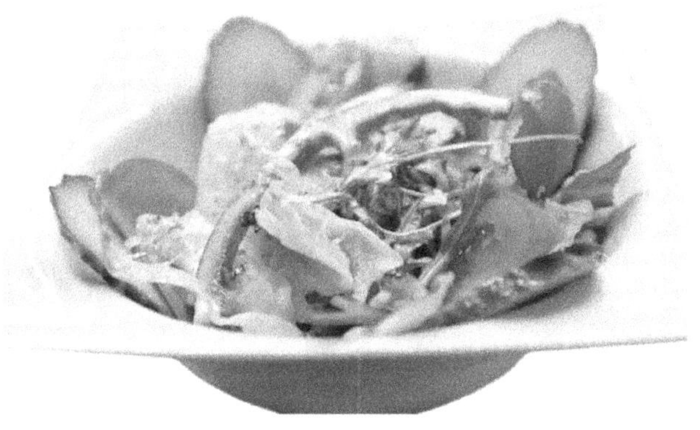

Dr. Malvin Harison

TABLE OF CONTENT

Introduction

Welcome to a culinary journey designed exclusively for you – a cherished senior seeking to embrace a vibrant and healthful life. In the pages that follow, we embark on a delicious exploration tailored to fortify your bones and enhance your overall well-being. This isn't just a cookbook; it's a companion on your path to combating osteoporosis through the joys of the kitchen.

In these recipes, we fuse simplicity with nutritional excellence, presenting a collection that not only tantalizes your taste buds but also supports bone health. Our aim is to make each meal a celebration of flavor and vitality, proving that a nourishing diet can be both easy to prepare and delightful to savor. Here's to a journey of health, happiness, and the joy of good food!

Overview of Osteoporosis

Osteoporosis is a condition characterized by a reduction in bone mineral density and mass, leading to weakened bone structure and an increased risk of fractures. It often goes unnoticed as it typically lacks noticeable symptoms until a bone is fractured. Postmenopausal women and older men are particularly susceptible, with fractures most commonly occurring in the hip, spine vertebrae, and wrist.

Causes of Osteoporosis

Osteoporosis is a condition characterized by weakened and porous bones, resulting from a loss of bone density. Several factors contribute to the development of osteoporosis, and understanding these causes is for prevention and management.

Here are some primary causes:

1. Aging: Aging is a significant factor in the development of osteoporosis. As we grow, density of bone naturally decreases, making bones more prone to fractures.

2. Hormonal Changes: Hormonal fluctuations, particularly a decrease in estrogen levels in women during menopause, can lead to accelerated bone loss. Similarly, reduced testosterone levels in men can also contribute to bone density decline.

3. Nutritional Deficiencies: Inadequate intake of calcium and vitamin D is a common cause of osteoporosis. Calcium is a key mineral for bone health, and vitamin D is essential for the absorption of calcium in the body.

4. Lack of Physical Activity: Sedentary lifestyles and lack of weight-bearing exercises can contribute to bone loss. Weight-bearing activities, such as walking, running, and weightlifting, stimulate bone formation and help maintain bone density.

5. Genetics: Genetic factors play a role in determining bone density. Individuals with a family history of osteoporosis may be more predisposed to developing the condition.

6. Medical Conditions: Certain medical conditions and treatments can increase the risk of osteoporosis. These include rheumatoid arthritis, celiac disease, and conditions that affect hormone levels.

7. Low Body Weight and Body Mass Index (BMI): People with low body weight or a low BMI may have less bone mass, making them more susceptible to osteoporosis.

8. Smoking and Excessive Alcohol Consumption: Smoking and excessive alcohol intake can contribute to bone loss. Smoking interferes with the absorption of calcium, while alcohol can interfere with the body's ability to use and absorb calcium.

Chapter 1:

The Importance of the Osteoporosis Diet Cookbook

1. Tailored Nutrition for Bone Health: The Osteoporosis Diet Cookbook is a treasure trove of recipes curated with your bone health in mind. Each dish is a carefully balanced masterpiece, rich in essential nutrients like calcium, vitamin D, protein, and other micronutrients vital for bone strength. It transforms meals into a proactive approach to fortify your bones from within.

II. Combatting Nutritional Deficiencies: Many seniors face challenges in maintaining optimal nutrient levels, especially calcium and vitamin D. This cookbook addresses these deficiencies head-on, offering delectable solutions that go beyond mere sustenance. It becomes your ally in ensuring that every bite contributes to the foundation of robust bones.

III. Empowering Through Choice: Variety is not just the spice of life; it's the cornerstone of a sustainable, healthful diet. The cookbook introduces you to a spectrum of flavors, textures, and culinary experiences. By making healthy eating enjoyable, it empowers you to make choices that support your well-being without compromising on the joy of food.

IV. Practicality Meets Healthfulness: We understand the need for simplicity. The recipes in this cookbook are designed for ease of preparation without sacrificing nutritional value.

Practicality becomes a guiding principle, making it accessible for everyone, regardless of culinary expertise.

V. Beyond the Plate: It's not just about what you eat; it's about how you nourish your entire lifestyle. The Osteoporosis Diet Cookbook extends beyond recipes, offering insights into meal planning, grocery shopping, and making informed choices when dining out. It's a holistic guide for embracing a bone-friendly lifestyle.

VI. A Culinary Journey to Resilience: This cookbook is more than ingredients and instructions; it's an invitation to embark on a culinary journey that celebrates life and health. Through vibrant flavors and nourishing meals, it transforms the act of eating into a deliberate, joyous step towards a stronger, more resilient you.

Complications of the Disease if the right diet is not taken

Choosing the right diet is like tending to the roots of a tree—essential for strength and resilience. In the realm of osteoporosis, neglecting this important aspect can set off a chain reaction of complications. Let's unravel the simple yet profound consequences of not nourishing your bones adequately.

1. Fragile Foundations: Without a diet rich in bone-supporting nutrients like calcium and vitamin D, your bones lose their sturdy foundation. This deficiency weakens them, making fractures and breaks more likely, turning the very structure of your body into fragile terrain.

2. Silent Struggles: Osteoporosis often creeps in unnoticed, silently eroding bone density.
A diet lacking in the right nutrients allows this silent struggle to persist,

escalating the risk of fractures without warning. It's like battling an invisible foe with an unarmed army.

3. Accelerated Decline: The absence of essential nutrients accelerates the natural aging process of your bones. Without proper nourishment, they succumb to rapid deterioration, robbing you of the strength and vitality needed for an active, fulfilling life.

4. Diminished Quality of Life: Imagine the joy of movement, the freedom to explore, and the confidence in your body's resilience. Without the right diet, these simple pleasures become compromised. Osteoporosis can limit your mobility and diminish your overall quality of life, turning once-enjoyable activities into potential sources of anxiety.

5. Increased Dependence: Fractures and bone-related issues can lead to increased dependence on others for daily activities. A diet lacking in bone-strengthening elements may inadvertently contribute to a loss of independence, as the risk of falls and injuries looms larger.

6. Pervasive Pain: Fragile bones often come hand-in-hand with persistent pain. Without the right nutrients, your bones struggle to repair and regenerate, leaving you vulnerable to chronic discomfort that permeates your daily life.

Foods to Eat for Strong Bones

1. Calcium-Rich Delights

a. Dairy: Milk, yogurt, and cheese are excellent sources of calcium. Opt for low-fat or non-fat varieties for a heart-healthy choice.

b. Leafy Greens: Embrace the power of greens like kale, spinach, and collard greens for a plant-based calcium boost.

2. Vitamin D Heroes

a. Fatty Fish: Salmon, mackerel, and tuna are not just delicious but also rich in vitamin D, a vital nutrient for calcium absorption.

b. Egg Yolks: The yolk is a natural source of vitamin D. Incorporate eggs into your diet in moderation.

3. Protein Powerhouses

a. Lean Proteins: Chicken, turkey, fish, beans, and lentils provide essential protein without the saturated fats found in some red meats.

b. Nuts and Seeds:* Almonds, chia seeds, and sunflower seeds contribute protein and other bone-boosting nutrients.

4. Whole Grains for Wholeness

a. Quinoa, Brown Rice, and Whole Wheat: These whole grains provide not only fiber but also essential minerals like magnesium, which supports bone health.

5. Fruits and Vegetables

a. Berries: Rich in antioxidants, berries contribute to overall health.

b. Oranges and Bell Peppers: These are excellent sources of vitamin C, which aids in collagen production, a key component of bone structure.

Foods to Limit or Avoid

1. Excessive Salt: High sodium intake can lead to calcium loss from the bones. Limit processed foods and opt for herbs and spices to flavor your meals.

2. Sugary Beverages: Soft drinks and sugary beverages can interfere with calcium absorption. Choose water, herbal teas, or milk as healthier alternatives.

3. Excessive Caffeine: While a moderate amount of caffeine is generally acceptable, excessive intake may interfere with calcium absorption. Balance your coffee or tea consumption with calcium-rich foods.

4. Alcohol in Excess: Excessive alcohol can interfere with the body's ability to absorb calcium. If you should drink, do it in moderation.

5. Highly Processed Foods: Processed foods often lack the nutritional value found in whole, natural foods.

Chapter 2: Nutrients-Rich Breakfast Recipes for Osteoporosis in seniors

1. Quinoa Breakfast Bowl

Ingredients
- 1/2 cup quinoa (rinsed)
- 1 cup almond milk
- 1 tablespoon chia seeds
- 1/2 cup mixed berries
- 1 tablespoon chopped nuts (almonds, walnuts)

Instructions
1. Cook quinoa in almond milk until it absorbs the liquid.
2. Stir in chia seeds and let it sit for 5 minutes.
3. Top with mixed berries and chopped nuts.

Serving: 1 serving

Nutritional Value

- Protein: 15g
- Calcium: 180mg
- Fiber: 8g
Cooking Time: 15 minutes

2. Greek Yogurt Parfait

Ingredients

- 1 cup Greek yogurt
- 1/2 cup granola (low-sugar)
- 1/4 cup sliced strawberries
- 1 tablespoon honey

Instructions

1. Turn Greek yogurt, granola, and strawberries into layers in a glass.
2. Drizzle honey on top.

Serving: 1 serving

Nutritional Value

- Protein: 20g
- Calcium: 300mg
- Vitamin D: 10% DV

Cooking Time: 5 minutes

3. Spinach and Feta Omelette

Ingredients

- 2 eggs
- 1 cup fresh spinach
- 2 tablespoons feta cheese (crumbled)
- 1/4 cup cherry tomatoes (halved)

Instructions

1. Whisk eggs and pour into a heated, oiled skillet.

2. Add spinach, feta, and tomatoes.

3. Fold the omelet and cook until eggs are set.

Serving: 1 serving

Nutritional Value

- Protein: 18g
- Calcium: 120mg
- Vitamin D: 6% DV

Cooking Time: 10 minutes

4. Salmon Avocado Toast

Ingredients

- 1 slice whole-grain bread
- 2 oz smoked salmon
- 1/2 avocado (sliced)
- 1 teaspoon lemon juice

Instructions

1. Toast the bread slice.

2. Top with smoked salmon and sliced avocado.

3. Drizzle with lemon juice.

Serving: 1 serving

Nutritional Value

- Protein: 15g
- Calcium: 80mg
- Omega-3 Fatty Acids

Cooking Time: 5 minutes

5. Chia Seed Pudding

Ingredients

- 2 tablespoons chia seeds
- 1 cup almond milk
- 1/2 teaspoon vanilla extract
- 1/4 cup mango chunks

Instructions

1. Mix chia seeds, almond milk, and vanilla extract.

2. Refrigerate overnight.

3. Top with mango chunks before serving.

Serving: 1 serving

Nutritional Value

- Protein: 10g

- Calcium: 220mg
- Fiber: 12g
Cooking Time: 10 minutes (plus overnight refrigeration)

6. Sweet Potato and Kale Breakfast Hash

Ingredients
- 1 medium sweet potato (diced)
- 1 cup kale (chopped)
- 2 eggs
- 1 tablespoon olive oil
- Salt and pepper to taste

Instructions
1. Sauté sweet potatoes in olive oil until golden brown.
2. Add chopped kale and cook until wilted.
3. Fry eggs and serve over the hash.

Serving: 1 serving

Nutritional Value
- Protein: 14g
- Calcium: 80mg
- Vitamin K: 400% DV

Cooking Time: 15 minutes

7. Cottage Cheese and Pineapple Bowl

Ingredients
- 1 cup low-fat cottage cheese
- 1/2 cup fresh pineapple (cubed)
- 1 tablespoon flax seeds
- 1 teaspoon honey

Instructions
1. Combine cottage cheese and pineapple.
2. Sprinkle with flaxseeds and drizzle with honey.

Serving: 1 serving

Nutritional Value
- Protein: 28g
- Calcium: 120mg
- Fiber: 4g

Cooking Time: 5 minutes

8. Whole Grain Pancakes with Blueberries

Ingredients

- 1/2 cup whole wheat flour
- 1/2 cup oat flour
- 1 teaspoon baking powder
- 1/2 cup almond milk
- 1 egg
- 1/2 cup blueberries

Instructions

1. Mix flours, baking powder, almond milk, and egg.
2. Cook pancakes on a griddle.
3. Top with fresh blueberries.

Serving: 2 servings

Nutritional Value

- Protein: 10g
- Calcium: 120mg
- Fiber: 6g

Cooking Time: 15 minutes

9. Mushroom and Spinach Breakfast Wrap

Ingredients

- 1 whole-grain tortilla
- 2 eggs (scrambled)
- 1/2 cup of mushrooms (sliced)

- 1 cup of fresh spinach
- 1 tablespoon of feta cheese

Instructions

1. Sauté mushrooms and spinach until wilted.

2. Scramble eggs and assemble the wrap with feta.

Serving: 1 serving

Nutritional Value

- Protein: 18g
- Calcium: 120mg
- Vitamin D: 8% DV

Cooking Time: 10 minutes

10. Pumpkin Pie Smoothie Bowl

Ingredients

- 1/2 cup canned pumpkin puree
- 1/2 banana
- 1/2 cup Greek yogurt
- 1/2 teaspoon pumpkin spice
- 1 tablespoon almond butter

Instructions

1. Blend pumpkin, banana, yogurt, pumpkin spice, and almond butter.
2. Pour into a bowl and add toppings of choice.

Serving: 1 serving

Nutritional Value

- Protein: 15g
- Calcium: 200mg
- Fiber: 5g

Cooking Time: 5 minutes

Chapter 3: Nutritious Lunch Recipes for Osteoporosis

Here are 10 nutrient-rich lunch recipes for the osteoporosis diet in seniors:

1. Salmon and Quinoa Salad

Ingredients

- 4 oz grilled salmon
- 1 cup cooked quinoa
- 1 cup mixed greens
- 1/2 cucumber (sliced)
- Cherry tomatoes (halved)

Instructions

1. Arrange mixed greens on a plate.
2. Top with quinoa, grilled salmon, cucumber, and cherry tomatoes.
3. Add with olive oil and lemon juice.

Serving: 1 serving

Nutritional Value

- Protein: 25g
- Calcium: 80mg
- Omega-3 Fatty Acids

Cooking Time: 20 minutes

2. Vegetable Stir-Fry with Tofu

Ingredients
- 1 cup tofu (cubed)
- Assorted vegetables (broccoli, bell peppers, carrots)
- 2 tablespoons soy sauce
- 1 tablespoon sesame oil

Instructions
1. Stir-fry tofu and vegetables in sesame oil.
2. Add soy sauce and cook until vegetables are tender.
3. Serve over brown rice.

Serving: 1 serving

Nutritional Value
- Protein: 20g
- Calcium: 150mg
- Fiber: 6g

Cooking Time: 15 minutes

3. Mediterranean Chickpea Salad

Ingredients

- 1 can chickpeas (drained)
- 1 cucumber (diced)
- 1 cup cherry tomatoes (halved)
- Feta cheese (crumbled)
- Kalamata olives (sliced)

Instructions

1. Mix chickpeas, cucumber, tomatoes, feta, and olives.
2. Spray with olive oil and balsamic vinegar.

Serving: 2 servings

Nutritional Value

- Protein: 12g
- Calcium: 100mg
- Fiber: 8g

Cooking Time: 10 minutes

4. Chicken and Broccoli Quiche

Ingredients

- 1 premade whole-grain pie crust
- 2 cups cooked chicken (shredded)
- 1 cup broccoli (steamed)
- 4 eggs
- 1 cup milk

Instructions:

1. Preheat the oven and bake pie crust.

2. Fill the crust with chicken and broccoli.

3. Whisk eggs and milk, pour over chicken and broccoli.

4. Bake until set.

Serving: 6 servings

Nutritional Value

- Protein: 18g
- Calcium: 120mg

Cooking Time: 30 minutes

5. Turkey and Avocado Wrap

Ingredients

- 1 whole-grain wrap
- 4 oz sliced turkey
- 1/2 avocado (sliced)
- Lettuce and tomato
- Greek yogurt spread

Instructions

1. Layer turkey, avocado, lettuce, and tomato on the wrap.
2. Spread with Greek yogurt.
3. Roll and slice.

Serving: 1 serving

Nutritional Value

- Protein: 20g
- Calcium: 100mg

Cooking Time: 10 minutes

6. Spinach and Lentil Soup

Ingredients

- 1 cup lentils (rinsed)
- 2 cups fresh spinach
- 1 onion (chopped)
- 2 carrots (sliced)

- 4 cups vegetable broth
Instructions
1. Sauté onion and carrots until softened.
2. Add lentils and vegetable broth; simmer until lentils are cooked.
3. Stir in fresh spinach before serving.
Serving: 4 servings
Nutritional Value
- Protein: 15g
- Calcium: 80mg
- Fiber: 12g
Cooking Time: 30 minutes

7. Eggplant and Chickpea Stew

Ingredients
- 1 eggplant (cubed)
- 1 can chickpeas (drained)
- 1 bell pepper (sliced)
- 1 can diced tomatoes
- 2 cloves garlic (minced)
Instructions
1. Sauté garlic, add eggplant, chickpeas, bell pepper, and tomatoes.
2. Simmer until vegetables are tender.

Serving: 3 servings
Nutritional Value
- Protein: 10g
- Calcium: 100mg
- Fiber: 8g
Cooking Time: 25 minutes

8. Shrimp and Asparagus Stir-Fry

Ingredients
- 1/2 lb shrimp (peeled and deveined)
- 1 bunch asparagus (trimmed)
- 1 bell pepper (sliced)
- 2 tablespoons low-sodium soy sauce
Instructions
1. Stir-fry shrimp, asparagus, and bell pepper.
2. Add soy sauce and cook until the shrimp are pink.
Serving: 2 servings
Nutritional Value
- Protein: 20g
- Calcium: 60mg
Cooking Time: 15 minutes

9. Tuna Salad Lettuce Wraps

Ingredients

- 1 can tuna (drained)
- 1/2 cup celery (chopped)
- 1/4 cup red onion (chopped)
- Greek yogurt
- Lettuce leaves

Instructions

1. Mix tuna, celery, and red onion with Greek yogurt.
2. Spoon into lettuce leaves for wraps.

Serving: 2 servings

Nutritional Value

- Protein: 15g
- Calcium: 60mg

Cooking Time: 10 minutes

10. Mushroom and Swiss Cheese Quinoa Bowl

Ingredients

- 1 cup cooked quinoa
- 1 cup mushrooms (sliced)
- 1 cup spinach
- 2 oz Swiss cheese (grated)

- 1 tablespoon olive oil

Instructions

1. Sauté mushrooms and spinach in olive oil.

2. Mix with cooked quinoa and top with Swiss cheese.

Serving: 1 serving

Nutritional Value

- Protein: 15g
- Calcium: 200mg

Cooking Time: 15 minutes

Chapter 4: Delicious dinner meals for seniors

Here are 10 delicious and nutrient-rich dinner recipes tailored for the osteoporosis diet:

1. Baked Salmon with Lemon-Dill Sauce

Ingredients
- 6 oz salmon filet
- 1 tablespoon olive oil
- 1 tablespoon fresh dill (chopped)
- 1 lemon (sliced)

Instructions
1. Place salmon on a baking sheet, drizzle with olive oil.
2. Sprinkle with chopped dill and lay lemon slices on top.
3. Bake until salmon flakes easily with a fork.

Serving: 1 serving

Nutritional Value
- Protein: 25g

- Calcium: 120mg
- Omega-3 Fatty Acids
Cooking Time: 20 minutes

2. Quinoa and Vegetable Stuffed Peppers

Ingredients
- 2 bell peppers (halved)
- 1 cup cooked quinoa
- 1 cup mixed vegetables (zucchini, cherry tomatoes, corn)
- 1/2 cup black beans (canned, rinsed)
Instructions
1. Roast bell peppers in the oven.
2. Mix cooked quinoa, vegetables, and black beans.
3. Stuff peppers with the mixture.
Serving: 2 servings
Nutritional Value
- Protein: 15g
- Calcium: 80mg
- Fiber: 8g
Cooking Time: 30 minutes

3. Chicken and Broccoli Brown Rice Bowl

Ingredients
- 1 cup cooked brown rice
- 4 oz grilled chicken breast (sliced)
- 1 cup broccoli (steamed)
- 1 tablespoon soy sauce

Instructions
1. Arrange brown rice, chicken, and broccoli in a bowl.
2. Mix with soy sauce.

Serving: 1 serving

Nutritional Value
- Protein: 30g
- Calcium: 100mg

Cooking Time: 20 minutes

4. Vegetarian Lentil Soup

Ingredients
- 1 cup dried lentils (rinsed)
- 1 onion (chopped)
- 2 carrots (sliced)
- 2 celery stalks (chopped)
- 4 cups vegetable broth

Instructions

1. Combine lentils, vegetables, and broth in a pot.
2. Simmer until lentils are tender.

Serving: 4 servings

Nutritional Value

- Protein: 18g
- Calcium: 80mg
- Fiber: 10g

Cooking Time: 30 minutes

5. Grilled Tofu Stir-Fry

Ingredients

- 1 cup firm tofu (cubed)
- Accompanied vegetable (bell peppers, broccoli, snap peas)
- 2 tablespoons low-sodium soy sauce
- 1 tablespoon sesame oil

Instructions

1. Grill tofu until golden.
2. Stir-fry tofu and vegetables in sesame oil.
3. Add soy sauce and cook until vegetables are tender.

Serving: 2 servings

Nutritional Value
- Protein: 20g
- Calcium: 150mg
- Fiber: 6g
Cooking Time: 20 minutes

6. Sweet Potato and Chickpea Curry

Ingredients
- 1 large sweet potato (diced)
- 1 can chickpeas (drained)
- 1 onion (chopped)
- 1 can diced tomatoes
- 2 tablespoons curry powder

Instructions
1. Sauté onion until softened, add sweet potato.
2. Stir in chickpeas, diced tomatoes, and curry powder.
3. Simmer until sweet potatoes are tender.
Serving: 3 servings
Nutritional Value
- Protein: 15g
- Calcium: 100mg
- Fiber: 8g

Cooking Time: 30 minutes

7. Whole Wheat Pasta with Spinach and Garlic

Ingredients

- 2 cups whole wheat pasta
- 2 cups fresh spinach
- 2 cloves garlic (minced)
- 2 tablespoons olive oil

Instructions

1. Cook pasta according to package instructions.
2. Sauté garlic in olive oil, add spinach and cooked pasta.
3. Toss until spinach wilts.

Serving: 2 servings

Nutritional Value

- Protein: 12g
- Calcium: 80mg

Cooking Time: 15 minutes

8. Turkey and Vegetable Skewers

Ingredients

- 8 oz turkey breast (cut into cubes)
- Assorted vegetables (bell peppers, cherry tomatoes, zucchini)
- 1 tablespoon olive oil
- 1 teaspoon Italian seasoning

Instructions

1. Thread turkey and vegetables onto skewers.
2. Drizzle with olive oil and sprinkle with Italian seasoning.
3. Grill until turkey is cooked through.

Serving: 2 servings

Nutritional Value

- Protein: 20g
- Calcium: 120mg

Cooking Time: 15 minutes

9. Egg Drop Soup with Vegetables

Ingredients
- 4 cups chicken or vegetable broth
- 2 eggs (beaten)
- 1 cup mixed vegetables (carrots, peas, corn)
- 2 green onions (sliced)

Instructions
1. Bring broth to a simmer, add mixed vegetables.
2. Slowly pour in beaten eggs, stirring gently.
3. Garnish with sliced green onions.

Serving: 2 servings

Nutritional Value
- Protein: 10g
- Calcium: 60mg

Cooking Time: 15 minutes

10. Baked Chicken and Sweet Potato

Ingredients
- 4 chicken thighs (bone-in, skin-on)
- 2 large sweet potatoes (sliced)
- 1 tablespoon olive oil

- 1 teaspoon paprika

Instructions

1. Preheat the oven and arrange chicken and sweet potatoes on a baking sheet.
2. Mizzle with olive oil and sprinkle with paprika.
3. Bake until chicken is cooked through and sweet potatoes are tender.

Serving: 2 servings

Nutritional Value

- Protein: 30g
- Calcium: 100mg

Cooking Time: 40 minutes

Chapter 5: Easy-to-prepare snacks and dessert

Here are 10 delicious and nutrient-rich snacks and dessert recipes for the osteoporosis diet:

1. Greek Yogurt with Berries

Ingredients
- 1 cup Greek yogurt
- 1/2 cup mixed berries (blueberries, strawberries)
- 1 tablespoon honey

Instructions
1. Spoon Greek yogurt into a bowl.
2. Top with mixed berries and drizzle with honey.

Serving: 1 serving

Nutritional Value
- Protein: 15g
- Calcium: 200mg
- Antioxidants from berries

2. Almond and Cheese Platter

Ingredients

- 1 oz almonds
- 1 oz cheese cubes (cheddar, mozzarella)
- 1/2 cup grapes

Instructions

1. Arrange almonds, cheese, and grapes on a plate.
2. Enjoy as a satisfying and balanced snack.

Serving: 1 serving

Nutritional Value

- Protein: 10g
- Calcium: 200mg
- Healthy fats from almonds

3. Hummus and Veggie Sticks

Ingredients

- 1/2 cup hummus
- Carrot and cucumber sticks
- Cherry tomatoes

Instructions

1. Dip veggie sticks into hummus.

2. Enjoy a crunchy and nutrient-rich snack.

Serving: 1 serving

Nutritional Value

- Protein: 8g
- Calcium: 60mg
- Fiber from veggies

4. Cottage Cheese and Pineapple

Ingredients

- 1/2 cup low-fat cottage cheese
- 1/2 cup pineapple chunks

Instructions

1. Combine cottage cheese and pineapple.

2. Enjoy a refreshing and protein-packed snack.

Serving: 1 serving

Nutritional Value

- Protein: 15g
- Calcium: 80mg
- Vitamin C from pineapple

5. Whole Grain Crackers with Tuna

Ingredients

- Whole grain crackers
- 1 can tuna (canned in water)
- 1 tablespoon Greek yogurt

Instructions

1. Mix tuna with Greek yogurt.
2. Spread on whole grain crackers for a satisfying snack.

Serving: 1 serving

Nutritional Value

- Protein: 15g
- Calcium: 40mg
- Omega-3 Fatty Acids

6. Baked Apples with Cinnamon

Ingredients

- 2 apples (cored and sliced)
- 1 teaspoon cinnamon
- 1 tablespoon honey

Instructions

1. Preheat the oven and place apple slices on a baking sheet.

2. Sprinkle with cinnamon and drizzle with honey.

3. Bake until the apples are tender.

Serving: 2 servings

Nutritional Value

- Fiber: 6g
- Antioxidants from apples
- Natural sweetness from honey

7. Chia Seed Pudding with Mango

Ingredients

- 2 tablespoons chia seeds
- 1 cup almond milk
- 1/2 teaspoon vanilla extract
- 1/2 cup diced mango

Instructions

1. Mix chia seeds, almond milk, and vanilla extract.

2. Refrigerate until a pudding-like consistency is achieved.

3. Top with diced mango before serving.

Serving: 1 serving

Nutritional Value

- Protein: 8g
- Calcium: 180mg

- Fiber: 12g

8. Dark Chocolate-Dipped Strawberries

Ingredients
- Dark chocolate (70% cocoa or higher)
- Fresh strawberries
Instructions
1. Melt dark chocolate in a bowl.
2. Dip each strawberry into the melted chocolate.
3. Place on a parchment-lined tray and refrigerate until the chocolate sets.
Serving: 1 serving
Nutritional Value
- Antioxidants from dark chocolate
- Vitamin C from strawberries

9. Yogurt Parfait with Granola and Berries

Ingredients
- 1 cup Greek yogurt
- 1/4 cup granola

- 1/2 cup mixed berries (blueberries, raspberries)

Instructions

1. Turn Greek yogurt, granola, and berries into layers in a glass.

2. Repeat the layers.

3. Enjoy a parfait-style dessert.

Serving: 1 serving

Nutritional Value

- Protein: 15g
- Calcium: 200mg
- Fiber from granola and berries

10. Frozen Banana Bites

Ingredients

- 2 bananas (peeled and sliced)
- 1/4 cup peanut butter
- 1/4 cup dark chocolate chips

Instructions

1. Spread peanut butter on banana slices and sandwich them together.

2. Dip each banana sandwich into melted dark chocolate.

3. Place on a tray and freeze until solid.

Serving: 2 servings

Nutritional Value

- Potassium from bananas
- Healthy fats from peanut butter
- Antioxidants from dark chocolate

Chapter 6: Bonus 1

7 days Sample Meal Plan

Day 1

Breakfast: Quinoa Breakfast Bowl.
Lunch: Greek Yogurt Parfait
Dinner: Baked Salmon with Lemon-Dill Sauce

Day 2:

Breakfast: Spinach and Feta Omelette
Lunch: Mediterranean Chickpea Salad
Dinner: Quinoa and Vegetable Stuffed

Day 3

Breakfast: Cottage Cheese and Pineapple Bowl
Lunch: Chicken and Broccoli Brown Rice Bowl
Dinner: Hummus and Veggie Sticks

Day 4

Breakfast: Whole Wheat Pancakes with Blueberries
Lunch: Tuna Salad Lettuce Wraps
Dinner: Turkey and Avocado Wrap

Day 5

Breakfast: Pumpkin Pie Smoothie Bowl
Lunch: Mushroom and Swiss Cheese Quinoa Bowl
Dinner: Baked Chicken and Sweet Potato

Day 6

Breakfast: Chia Seed Pudding with Mango
Lunch: Egg Drop Soup with Vegetables
Dinner: Shrimp and Asparagus Stir-Fry

Day 7

Breakfast: Sweet Potato and Chickpea Curry
Lunch: Vegetable Stir-Fry with Tofu
Dinner: Dark Chocolate-Dipped Strawberries

Chapter 7: Bonus 2

20 juicing and smoothie recipes for Osteoporosis

Here are 20 short and unique juicing and smoothie recipes for osteoporosis:

1. Calcium Greens Burst

Ingredients: Kale, spinach, cucumber.
Instructions: Juice all ingredients.
Serving: 1
Nutritional Value: Rich in calcium, vitamin K.
Cooking Time: 5 minutes

2. Citrus Collagen Kick

Ingredients: Oranges, grapefruit, cucumber.
Instructions: Juice and enjoy!
Serving: 1
Nutritional Value: Vitamin C for bone health.
Cooking Time: 3 minutes

3. Mango Tango Magnesium Mix

Ingredients: Mango, banana, spinach.
Instructions: Blend into a smoothie.
Serving: 1
Nutritional Value: Magnesium-rich.
Cooking Time: 5 minutes

4. Beetroot Bliss Booster

Ingredients: Beets, carrots, apples.
Instructions: Juice for a nutrient-packed elixir.
Serving: 1
Nutritional Value: Folate and manganese.
Cooking Time: 4 minutes

5. Ginger Gold Elixir

Ingredients: Ginger, apple, lemon.
Instructions: Juice for an anti-inflammatory blend.
Serving: 1
Nutritional Value: Ginger's anti-inflammatory properties.
Cooking Time: 3 minutes

6. Bone Berry Burst

Ingredients: Mixed berries, Greek yogurt, almond milk.
Instructions: Blend into a delicious smoothie.
Serving: 1
Nutritional Value: Calcium and vitamin D.
Cooking Time: 5 minutes

7. Tropical Twist Delight

Ingredients: Pineapple, mango, coconut water.
Instructions: Blend for a tropical treat.
Serving: 1
Nutritional Value: Potassium and magnesium.
Cooking Time: 4 minutes

8. Avocado Almond Bliss

Ingredients: Avocado, almonds, and bananas.

Instructions: Blend for a creamy delight.
Serving: 1
Nutritional Value: Healthy fats and potassium.
Cooking Time: 5 minutes

9. Spinach Citrus Surge

Ingredients: Spinach, orange, banana.
Instructions: Blend into a green powerhouse.
Serving: 1
Nutritional Value: Vitamin K and antioxidants.
Cooking Time: 4 minutes

10. Papaya Passion Potion

Ingredients: Papaya, pineapple, coconut milk.
Instructions: Blend for a tropical sip.
Serving: 1
Nutritional Value: Vitamin C and calcium.
Cooking Time: 4 minutes

11. Cucumber Mint Cooler

Ingredients: Cucumber, mint, lime.
Instructions: Blend for a refreshing treat.
Serving: 1
Nutritional Value: Hydrating and bone-friendly.
Cooking Time: 3 minutes

12. Blueberry Basil Bliss

Ingredients: Blueberries, basil, yogurt.
Instructions: Blend for a unique flavor.
Serving: 1
Nutritional Value: Antioxidants and calcium.
Cooking Time: 4 minutes

13. Carrot Kale Glow

Ingredients: Carrots, kale, orange.
Instructions: Juice for a vibrant concoction.
Serving: 1

Nutritional Value: Beta-carotene and vitamin C.
Cooking Time: 4 minutes

14. Turmeric Citrus Crush

Ingredients: Turmeric, oranges, ginger.
Instructions: Juice for an anti-inflammatory burst.
Serving: 1
Nutritional Value: Turmeric's anti-inflammatory properties.
Cooking Time: 3 minutes

15. Pear Basil Refresher

Ingredients: Pears, basil, cucumber.
Instructions: Juice for a unique flavor twist.
Serving: 1
Nutritional Value: Rich in vitamins and minerals.
Cooking Time: 4 minutes

16. Cranberry Kale Quencher

Ingredients: Cranberries, kale, and apples.
Instructions: Juice for a tangy kick.
Serving: 1
Nutritional Value: Vitamin C and antioxidants.
Cooking Time: 3 minutes

17. Pomegranate Paradise

Ingredients: Pomegranate seeds, spinach, cucumber.
Instructions: Juice for a refreshing treat.
Serving: 1

Nutritional Value: Antioxidants and vitamin K.
Cooking Time: 4 minutes

18. Broccoli Banana Boost

Ingredients: Broccoli, banana, almond milk.
Instructions: Blend for a nutrient-packed smoothie.
Serving: 1
Nutritional Value: Calcium and vitamin C.
Cooking Time: 5 minutes

19. Minty Pineapple Pleasure

Ingredients: Pineapple, mint, Greek yogurt.
Instructions: Blend for a tropical and refreshing delight.
Serving: 1
Nutritional Value: Calcium and digestive benefits.
Cooking Time: 4 minutes

20. Cherry Vanilla Dream

Ingredients: Cherries, vanilla protein powder, almond milk.

Instructions: Blend for a tasty protein-packed smoothie.

Serving: 1

Nutritional Value: Protein, calcium, and antioxidants.

Cooking Time: 4 minutes

Conclusion

Embracing a bone-healthy lifestyle doesn't mean sacrificing flavor; it's about savoring the vibrant fusion of nutrients that nourish and fortify. Here's to your well-balanced journey towards stronger bones and a tastier tomorrow! Cheers to a life filled with delicious wellness!